Table of Contents

Introduction 5

Chapter 1. Main Principles of Fasting Diet 6

Chapter 2. How Fasting Diet Helps in Weight Loss and Provides Healthy Living 7

Chapter 3. Foods to Eat and Foods to Avoid 10

Chapter 4. Fasting Diet Food Plan 14

    Meal Plan 1: Less Than 900 Total Calories 14

    Meal Plan 2: Less Than 1000 Total Calories 16

Chapter 5. Fasting Diet Recipes 18

    1. Breakfast Recipes 18

    2. Lunch and Dinner Recipes 21

    3. Snack Recipes 24

Conclusion 27

Thank You Page 29

Fasting Diet For Beginners: Easy and Fast Dieting Tips For Weight Loss and Healthy Living

By Brittany Samons

© Copyright 2014 Brittany Samons

Reproduction or translation of any part of this work beyond that permitted by section 107 or 108 of the 1976 United States Copyright Act without permission of the copyright owner is unlawful. Requests for permission or further information should be addressed to the author.

This publication is designed to provide accurate and authoritative information in regard to the subject matter covered. This work is sold with the understanding that the publisher is not engaged in rendering legal, accounting, or other professional services. If legal advice or other expert assistance is required, the services of a competent professional person should be sought.

First Published, 2014

Printed in the United States of America

Introduction

A fasting diet is basically indulging in a diet plan that limits the amount of calories that you take in a day. It may also be a diet that completely prohibits eating anything just like what the name suggests. But since it is impossible even for a healthy person to not eat anything and still function at home and at work, proponents of countless fasting diet versions have come up with their best approaches to fasting. One such method is fasting intermittently.

Intermittent fasting is eating less than the amount of calories that you usually take in a day while eating the usual way in some days. Another way to start a fasting diet is to gradually indulge in it instead of jumping into a straightforward fast. An intermittent diet plan is wherein you must fast or limit your meals to only 500 calories in a day for 2 non-consecutive days while you eat your usual diet for the rest of the days of the week. People that have actually tried the an intermittent plan agree that this is one of the best ways to lose weight especially for those who are new to fasting and also it has a lot of health benefits as well.

Chapter 1. Main Principles of Fasting Diet

The principles of a fasting diet is to reduce your weight by reducing the amount of calories that you take in. it is reasonable enough that if a person would like to reduce his weight or to achieve his ideal weight for his age and his height then he should limit the amount of calories that he should take in a day. By doing so, he will be able to eventually manage a feasible diet that could help him lose weight.

But of course indulging in a fasting diet should be done in an idealistic manner. Not everyone may use this kind of diet basically not all people are alike. Healthy individuals may use fasting to lose weight and may even fast for two or more days to achieve their goals however there are some people such as diabetics, people with nutritional deficiencies, people with intolerance to certain foods, pregnant and breastfeeding women and other people that have medical conditions are not advised to fast or indulge in a fasting diet.

If you plan to use a fasting diet or an intermittent fasting diet then you should consult your doctor beforehand. You may also consult a dietician or a nutritionist to help you develop a fasting diet plan.

Chapter 2. How Fasting Diet Helps in Weight Loss and Provides Healthy Living

Fasting is beneficial to the body in many ways but only to some extent. This is why consulting a doctor or a medical professional before indulging in a fasting diet is essential

1. Fasting diet can help detoxify the body. A kind of fasting diet is eating only fruits and vegetables since these kinds of foods are known to contain only a few calories and are very filling. You are least likely to crave for food in between meals when you eat fruits and veggies and you may also be able to avoid overeating as well. Veggies and fruits are also known to contain fibre which is found in ruminants of vegetables and in the skins and meat of fruits. Fiber cleanses the body by removing toxins and microorganisms that may cause diseases in the gut. Fiber also regulates your colon enabling you to move your bowels regularly as well.

2. Fasting diet helps prevent various diseases related to obesity and being overweight. It is known that there are so many diseases that a person with obesity is likely to suffer. Aside from hypertension, an overweight person may also be able to avoid increased cholesterol levels, diabetes, arthritis and cardiovascular diseases. When a fasting diet is efficiently

done, an obese person may be able to reduce his weight in the safest and the most effective manner possible and of course avoid these dangerous medical conditions.

3. Intermittent fasting diet induces a "repair mode" which is a complete opposite of storing fat or "starvation mode." The body restores cells that have been damaged due to fasting and restoring cells needs energy. The longer you safely fast the more the body is in repair mode and hence you are able to lose weight in the process.

4. Fasting and intermittent fasting helps in weight loss since it is very easy to remember and hence is very easy to use. It is unlike diets that require you to count calories, read product labels and compute important figures to comply with a meal plan. The fasting diet is challenging to do but relatively easy to implement. Simply put, the less you eat the more weight that you are likely to lose.

5. Finally a fasting diet like the intermittent fasting diet is flexible and thus will help a person that would like to lose weight. By complying with an intermittent fasting diet, you will be able to lose weight and maintain a healthy body without impacting your health. You can fast during the weekends when you need fewer calories since you are resting and relaxing at home. And of course you are allowed to eat

the meals that you enjoy during the weekdays when you are likely to need more energy with all the activities that you do during these days.

Chapter 3. Foods to Eat and Foods to Avoid

As mentioned, the fasting diet is very easy to follow. When it comes to the foods that you must eat and those that you must avoid, there is actually no such rule. All you need is to stick to your allowed calories in a day. For instance, females require 1500 to 2000 calories in a day while males need 2000 to 2500 calories. A fasting diet may require you to take only half of your allowable calorie intake therefore you can eat anything provided you stay within the range.

But of course even with this obvious restriction, a person that uses a fasting diet should be aware of foods that have high calorie content as well as foods that have hidden calories. You must avoid the following foods:

1. Animal fats should be avoided or limited in your diet. Animal fats are high in saturated fats and cholesterol and are also very high in calories. Lard and fish oils have 902 calories per 100 grams while butter contains 876 calories per 100 gram serving.

2. Vegetable oils such as peanut oil, palm oil and soybean oil are also known to have high calorie content. These oils have 884 calories per 100 gram serving. Just to translate into actual serving sizes that you may recognize a cup of vegetable

oil has 1927 calories, a tablespoon has 124 calories and a teaspoon as 44 calories.

3. Salad dressings also have high calories and to think that you must have indulged in eating fresh vegetable salads to lose weight. French dressings have 631 calories per 100 grams and runner ups are Caesar's salad dressing, ranch dressing and blue cheese salad dressing.

4. Junk foods are loaded with calories as well as salt and fat. There are so many types of junk foods but the usual kind may have anywhere to 500 or more calories per 100 grams serving. Traditional junk foods like candy bars contain 260 calories while the most common cheese puff junk food variety may contain more than 1200 calories.

5. Fried foods also contain the highest calories since aside from the actual food that you eat the oil that was also used to fry the food also adds to the list. Fried chicken contains 460 calories per 100 grams, French fries have 370 calories per 100 grams serving and onion rings contain 407 calories per 100 grams.

6. Cheeses especially parmesan and the Norwegian Brunost contain the most calories. The Brunost has 466 calories per 100 gram serving.

7. Dark chocolate, although has amazing amounts of antioxidants, contain a lot of calories. Baking chocolate contains 501 calories.

And if there is a long line of foods that you should never eat while you are in a fasting diet there is also a huge list of low calorie foods that you may eat while you indulge in this kind of diet.

1. Berries are the top of the list since a cup of berries only has 85 calories. You may eat berries like blueberries, strawberries and blackberries on their own, place them in a cup and chill for dessert or may be added to cereal in the morning.

2. Eggs are perfect for a fasting diet since a large egg contains 70 to 80 calories only. You may boil or poach eggs but do not fry eggs since you will only add more calories to your meals.

3. Broccoli contains only 95 calories per cup and this number includes a 3 tablespoon low calorie dip of your choice.

4. An apple with its peel contains only 70 calories. Apples are also filling since most of its weight is water. A known fasting diet is the apple diet wherein the dieter only eats apples as much as he can in a day or drinks only apple juice.

5. Kiwis have the lowest calories with only 95 calories for two medium sized fruit. So indulge in sweet kiwi for snacks or as a lunch time dessert.

6. Whole grain bread has only 65 calories per slice. This is why whole grain breads are used in low fat sandwiches and in preparing low calorie breakfast meals.

7. Light beer has only 95 calories per 12 fl. oz. bottle. So there is no reason to forget your favourite pastime when you are on a fasting diet. Be sure to drink moderately.

8. Baked or broiled salmon at 2 ½ oz. contains only 99 calories so therefore it is a great idea to serve salmon during main meals when you are on a fasting diet.

9. Watermelon contains fewer calories compared to other fruits and is also a great source of water. 2 cups of watermelon contains only 90 calories.

10. A skinless chicken drumstick only contains 75 calories but when you leave the skin on will double its calorie amount! Chicken meat prepared using other methods other than deep frying are also known to have fewer calories.

Chapter 4. Fasting Diet Food Plan

A fasting diet food plan is very easy to visualize when you understand how a particular fasting diet plan goes. As mentioned, the most popular fasting diet is the intermittent fasting wherein the dieter limits the amount of calories that he takes in for two non-consecutive days of the week while he keeps to his usual diet or meals during the rest of the week. If this is considered, here is what an actual fasting diet meal plan looks like:

For a dieter that is required to take only 1000 calories for a fasting day

Meal Plan 1: Less Than 900 Total Calories

Breakfast

¾ cup of skimmed milk at 68 calories

1/3 cups of rolled oats at 93 calories

½ apple at 47 calories

A glass of water at 0 calories

Snacks

A cup of blue berries at 85 calories

Lunch

Scrambled eggs at 72 calories for the egg and 11 calories for a tablespoon of fat-free milk

A slice of whole wheat bread at 70 calories

½ oz. of cheddar cheese at 25 calories

Snacks

A bowl of almonds at 90 calories

Dinner

3 oz. chicken breast at 142 calories

For a salad: 2 cups of shredded lettuce at 10 calories, 6 cherry tomatoes at 30 calories, ½ cups of sliced red pepper at 12 calories, a thinly sliced red online at 48 calories and a tablespoon of low-fat salad dressing at 24 calories

Meal Plan 2: Less Than 1000 Total Calories

Breakfast

A whole wheat muffin at 120 calories

A pat of butter at 36 calories

A cup of fruit at 74 calories

A glass of water or tea

Snacks

A cup of watermelons at 45 calories

Lunch

Tuna salad with the following ingredients: a chopped apple with 94 calories, 3 oz. of tuna in water at 99 calories, 2 cups of romaine lettuce leaves at only 10 calories and a tablespoon of low fat mayonnaise at 45 calories.

¼ cup of plain low fat yoghurt at only 36 calories

Snacks

A cup of air popped popcorn at 31 calories

Dinner

4 ounces of chicken breast, grilled with no skin at 189 calories

A small tossed green salad with two tablespoons of dressing at 61 calories

A cup of green beans at 44 calories

A small spread of butter on your beans at only 36 calories.

Chapter 5. Fasting Diet Recipes

1. Breakfast Recipes

Cold Breakfast Smoothie

Choose the kind of fruit that you wish to eat or rather drink; you may use strawberries, raspberries or bananas depending on what fruit is in season. You will need about 5 strawberries with the hulls removed, half a ripe banana and about 200 ml of ice cold skimmed milk. Place all the ingredients in a blender and then blend till the ingredients are smooth. You may even add crushed ice to make it a more pleasing drink.

Bacon, Eggs and Tomato

This breakfast treat is easy to make and contains only a number of calories. You will need 2 reduce fat bacon strips, a large-size egg, a tomato cut in half and a light spray of sunflower oil for frying.

Use a large frying pan and prepare it by placing it on medium heat before cooking the ingredients. Use a fine spray of sunflower oil so that you will be able to prevent the ingredients from sticking. Cook the bacon and then the tomato halves for about 3 minutes. Keep turning the bacon and the tomato halves until these are cooked. When these are ready, crack open the egg into the pan and then cook for another five minutes. When the egg hardens this means that the dish is ready to be served.

Salmon and Cheese for Breakfast

This recipe is a bit time consuming to prepare but you can do this the night before. You will need a 2 tablespoons of light cheese, freshly squeezed half lemon, dash of freshly ground black pepper, 2 ½ oz. of salmon cut in small sizes and a lemon wedge as an ornament.

Place the cheese, lemon juice and pepper in a small bowl. Mix well. Set the dish with two pieces of salmon in cross shape. Place cream cheese in the middle of the cross and then bring the sides of the fish towards the top and secure with a toothpick. Create a parcel of all the salmon that you have and then place in a dry container with a cover and refrigerate. You may also eat this once it is done; place a lemon wedge on the side of the plate as you eat.

Delicious Courgette and Eggs Breakfast

This is a breakfast omelette made from courgette and chives. It is easy to prepare and has very simple ingredients too. You will need a courgette, 2 medium-sized eggs, and a teaspoon of chives and a dash of olive oil. Grate the courgette and then chop the chives. Mix all these in a small bowl and then place a drop of olive oil in a medium-sized pan. Place the mixture in the pan as soon as it is hot. Cook well on each side and then serve immediately.

2. Lunch and Dinner Recipes

Honey and Mustard Chicken

You will need to marinate this chicken for about 30 minutes so that it will come out tasting very tender. It is recommended that you serve this honey and mustard chicken in a skewer with green salad. You will need 2 tablespoons of wholegrain mustard, a teaspoon of honey, zest of lime and one 150 g chicken without skin. Prepare the chicken by cutting into small pieces, mix the honey, mustard, lime and juice in a bowl. Place the chicken in the mixture and then coat the chicken with the mixture completely. Marinate this for about 30 minutes to an hour.

Preheat your grill and then place the marinated chicken in skewers. Place the chicken on the grill when the grill is ready and then grill the chicken for 8 minutes on each side. Check on the chicken as it grills to prevent charring it. Baste the chicken with the marinade as regularly as you can. Serve this with or without the skewers.

Chicken Fillets with Feta Cheese

This is a tasty chicken dish that is also very low in calories. You need 150g chicken fillets, a tablespoon of tomato paste, a teaspoon of fresh basil chopped a teaspoon of olive oil, a clove of garlic sliced into small pieces, a dash of salt, a tablespoon of red wine and 25g of feta cheese (light). Prepare the cheese by cutting these into very small cubes. Prepare the chicken fillet by cutting it into two pieces and then scoring the fillets on each side. Combine the tomato paste and half the chopped fresh basil on the chicken pieces; after basting the chicken with tomato paste and basil, set it aside. Take a non-stick pan of medium size; heat the oil and then sauté the garlic in it until it is colored brown. Add the tomatoes, the remaining basil leaves and salt. Cook for another 10 minutes. Break open the tomatoes and then add the red wine. Continue cooking the dish for another 10 minutes. Heat up your grill to medium heat and then when it is ready place the chicken on the grill. Cook the chicken fillet pieces for about 7 minutes on each side; the chicken is cooked when its sides are golden brown. When the chicken is ready, add this to the tomato sauce mixture and then add the feta cheese. Stir everything and cook for another 3 minutes and then remove from heat.

Tiger Prawns in a Barbecue

This is a low calorie dish that is perfect for dinner or lunch time since 8 oz. of prawns only has 171 calories. You will need about 225 g of tiger prawns and freshly squeezed lemon juice. For the shrimp marinade you will need 2 cloves of garlic, zest of lemon, a tablespoon of olive oil, a teaspoon of fresh parsley and salt and pepper to taste.

Prepare the parsley and the garlic cloves by chopping these into fine pieces. Make the marinade by combining all the marinade ingredients in a bowl. Clean and place the shrimps in the marinade for 30 minutes to an hour. Preheat the grill in medium heat. Grill the tiger prawns for 2 to 3 minutes on each side and then turning these frequently to cook. When the prawns are cooked, place these on a tray and then squeeze the lemon over them. Serve immediately afterwards. If you should serve this meal later, do not place lemon juice over the shrimps yet. Allow your shrimps to stay on the top most level of your grill and then bring them back to the flame if you are ready to serve.

3. Snack Recipes

Cold Fruit Fiesta Cups

Fruits like berries and melons are lowest in calories plus will also make you feel fuller to avoid snacking in between meals. This is a very easy recipe that you need to prepare beforehand so you can serve or eat this chilled.

You will need any fruit in season like melons, apples, pineapples and berries to name few. You will also need small plastic cups. Cut the melon and with the use of a melon baller too, scoop a few balls and then place these into the cups. Allow the skin on the apple to remain and then cut these into cubes or bite-sized pieces. Pineapples may be bought in a can or you may prepare your own pineapple tidbits by cutting these into very small pieces. Berries may be washed and then any top part removed. Place each fruit in the cups provided and chill these. Do not place any cream or sugar since this will only add more calories to your snacks.

Crunchy Veggies

As mentioned before, fruits and vegetables are great candidates for the fasting diet since these contain very little calories and have high amounts of fibre. Therefore the best snack for a fasting diet is to eat vegetables, the crunchy variety.

Prepare 2 celery stalks, a medium sized cucumber, a medium sized carrot and a red bell pepper. Wash the celery stalks and remove any leaves; cut these to about two inches long and set these aside in a small bowl. Cut the cucumber with skin into small pieces about the size of the celery stalks. Remove the skin of the carrot and the top part and then cut these into the size of the celery stalks. The red bell peppers will also need to be cut the same way but remove seeds. Arrange these in a small platter with a low calorie dip in the middle.

Fruit Snack Smoothies

Fruit smoothies are not just perfect for breakfast but it also works as the perfect snack food.

You need a cup of pineapples, chopped ripe bananas and melons. Simply cut all the ingredients into small pieces and then place in a blender; blend the fruits with crushed ice. You may add ½ cup of almond milk to the mixture and then blend for another minute. Serve your fruit smoothies in a tall glass with a large straw.

Cheese and Crackers Snacks

A saltine low salt cracker only has 13 calories and a couple of these won't hurt your fasting diet along with a slice of Asda Cheese light with only 38 calories. You will need two Saltine crackers and a couple of slices of Asda cheese. Simply place a slice of cheese over a saltine cracker and then eat. You may also place a drizzle of olive oil over your cheese for more flavour.

Conclusion

A fasting diet could be considered as a replacement of your usual meal however since most of these meal plans contain very little calories it is very important to reconsider if this is really the ideal weight loss diet to use. And since there are reduced nutrients that are taken by the body, the need to use supplements is often considered to augment a low calorie diet such as a fasting diet.

And aside from lacking nutrients that can lead to medical conditions, fasting diets may even lead to rebound in the end. As they say the more you prohibit eating foods that a person or dieter is used to, she will only crave more and thus results to overeating and an increased weight after a significant weight loss happens. Therefore any kind of diet that involves a drastic change in the eating habits of a person should be dealt through a better and a safer manner.

Diet should be accompanied by exercise. But how will a person that has been significantly cutting down on calories may withstand the rigors of exercise. Therefore, still the best way to find a more suitable exercise plan despite eating a very low calorie diet should be endorsed to a professional trainer or gym instructor beforehand. You should also never take any weight loss supplements despite great news about how effective and efficient supplements are. Following a fasting diet meal combined with the ideal exercise plan and doing away with bad health and eating habits could help save your wellness in the long run. And so are fasting diets worthy to be called radical diets? In essence it is very hard to commit to a fasting diet especially when you need a lot of calories for energy for all your many activities throughout the day. Therefore a close assessment of your calorie needs and physical activity will be at hand before indulging in this diet.

Thank You Page

I want to personally thank you for reading my book. I hope you found information in this book useful and I would be very grateful if you could leave your honest review about this book. I certainly want to thank you in advance for doing this.

www.ingramcontent.com/pod-product-compliance
Lightning Source LLC
LaVergne TN
LVHW021946060526
838200LV00042B/1934